# JOURNEY THROUGH CANCER

First published 1993

This edition published 2010
Veritas Publications
7–8 Lower Abbey Street
Dublin 1, Ireland
Email publications@veritas.ie
Website www.veritas.ie

ISBN 978 1 84730 211 3

10 9 8 7 6 5 4 3 2 1

A catalogue record for this book is available from the
British Library.

Printed in Ireland by ColourBooks Ltd, Dublin

Veritas books are printed on paper made from the wood
pulp of managed forests. For every tree felled, at least one
tree is planted, thereby renewing natural resources.

# JOURNEY THROUGH CANCER

JEAN LAVELLE

VERITAS

# CONTENTS

# PREFACE

This book is about a healing process. It is about the painful business of maturing.

There are umpteen different forms of cancer and the causes of most of them are unknown. There is scarcely a family today that has not been touched by cancer in some way. We all know or have heard of someone who has had cancer, but when you are told you have cancer, what do you do? You can try to hold on until the researchers discover the cause and the cure for it, but maybe there are as many causes as there are patients! What then? This is the story of what I did. That is all. I make no claims and I hope I make no generalisations. But maybe what I have to say will help someone else in their struggle with the disease.

I chose to see the cancer I had as something very personal to me. Having had surgery for it twice, I realised that I must assume responsibility for my own life and everything in it. That is, I decided that I must respond to the cancer – not by making a frantic search for a cure outside myself, not by waiting for the dreaded disease to recur, but by journeying towards healing inside myself. My journey has not been easy but it has been worthwhile.

No two people are the same; no two people will respond to cancer in the same way. I am sharing my journey with you so that if there is something in it that will resonate with you, then it may help you along your way.

When you have overcome cancer you are indebted to a multitude of people. I want to thank my husband for the enormous support he gave me throughout the illness. Without him I would have gone under. I thank him too for his support in the writing of this account, which he has read at all its stages. Without him it would not have seen the light of day.

I want to thank the doctors, the nurses and the hospital staff. I want to thank all those people who helped me (some of whom will recognise themselves here, despite name changes), and the many, known and unknown, who prayed for me.

Names have been altered to preserve anonymity and privacy, but everything is told as it happened.

Finally, I thank Fr Nivard, monk of Mount St Joseph Abbey, Roscrea, for his enthusiasm for the project of writing it all down and for his help in doing so.

## A DAY TO REMEMBER – A DAY TO FORGET

It was the end of August and I was flying around in the whole of my health (as I thought) with only three things on my mind: have a new hair-do – a body-wave! – bring the children to the seaside for a day, and buy them their school uniforms. Then, like a bird shot down in mid-flight, my life changed.

For four years I had had a black spot in my left thumbnail. I always thought that I must have caught it in something, like a door, to have caused the injury. But I had no memory of injuring it. Having a very young family to care for I knew that there were days when I could have caught my head in a door and not noticed! When bringing the children to various doctors for minor ailments over the years, I showed the nail. The doctors invariably made nothing of it. Indeed one of them cheerfully told me to put nail varnish on it!

Eventually a doctor said to me, 'If I were you, Jean, I would show that nail to a surgeon. I think maybe he might take it off and it would grow clean again.' I had wondered myself how the black spot had not grown out of the nail. No blame to the doctors – most doctors would never in a lifetime come across malignant melanoma of the nail tissue. So I finally went to a surgeon who did a biopsy. My husband Jim was with me in the waiting room when I went to get the result. The surgeon came in and, standing in front of me, said in a grave voice: 'The news is not good. It is cancer.'

My immediate reaction was to sway to and fro in the chair and repeat in a loud whisper, 'I'm having a nightmare – I'll come out of it.' My husband managed to remain calm, and placing his hand on my left shoulder, communicated some of that calm to me. I felt as if an earthquake was taking place in the very pit of my being. If only I could wake up and discover that I was having one hell of a nightmare, but my sanity would not allow me to escape this cruel reality. I had cancer. Or rather, it had me! The surgeon went on to suggest amputation of the whole thumb, which he would perform the next morning. My husband thanked him and told him we needed a few hours to think about it. As we stood up to leave, my legs felt like jelly, while the rest of my body was numb. My husband linked me out to the car where our children were waiting to be brought shopping for their school uniforms. We explained that we could not go shopping that day. They did not protest. They were silent and were not fooled by our efforts to hide our shock. Silent tears flowed. The day you are told you have cancer is a day to remember in order to forget.

Inwardly I felt as if I was a babe again, back in my mother's womb. From a distance I could overhear that I was to die before the time was ripe for me to be born, before the time was ripe for me to make conscious contact with my own creative centre, get a sense of my real self. I felt engulfed by a feeling of quiet desperation.

When we got home we phoned an old schoolfriend of mine who is a nun and also a theatre nurse. Sr Mary said she would phone me back within an hour or so when, hopefully, she would have made arrangements for me to see another surgeon.

Then I flopped down into a two-seater in our kitchen, feeling as if my heart was breaking. Our nine-year-old son, Anthony, disappeared into his bedroom to cry. Always a sensitive child, he could not look at anyone in pain. After a while he returned to the kitchen looking so calm and peaceful that I was astonished. I know him and I wondered what had happened. He had run away from me in fear to cry and be alone. Now he appeared to have lost all fear and wanted to draw close to me. He moved slowly and, sitting down beside me, he hugged me, opened his hand and showed me a Green Scapular of Our Lady. He then explained with the disarming simplicity and faith of a child that when he was lying on his bed crying he had remembered the Green Scapular under his pillow. He reached in for it and at the very moment he held it in his hand, a little shock went right through him, which conveyed to him, 'Your Mammy is going to be all right.'

It was obvious from the child's whole countenance and demeanour that he was grounded in a truth too great for me to comprehend in my present state of bewilderment. It was wonderful to be hugged by a child whose overwhelming fear had been transformed into a peace beyond all understanding.

Then the phone rang. It was Mary to say that she had made arrangements for me to see another surgeon next morning. My husband and I felt somewhat easier now that we were going to have a second opinion.

Next morning the second surgeon confirmed the diagnosis, but said that amputation of the thumb from the first joint would be sufficient to deal with the condition. I felt relieved on hearing this news. Then I asked the surgeon if the rest of the thumb might have to be amputated later should the cancer return. He said, 'No! The form of cancer you have is only interested in nail tissue.' I was not offered chemotherapy or radium treatment, 'as research shows that the cancer you have would not respond to such treatment'. The surgeon went on to give me some statistics about the likelihood of my being alive in one year, two years and so on. By the time the surgeon mentioned the fifth year there were no statistics left. I got the message. My term of office on this earth would be up within five years. It sounded very like a death sentence, but I was so relieved at losing only half my thumb that I let the statistics in one ear and out the other. A few days later I was on the operating table.

## A PROVIDENTIAL MEETING

Several years before I knew I had cancer, I came across an article written by Fr Robert Nash SJ, entitled 'Is it Cancer?' I decided to keep it, as I thought one could get great consolation from reading the article if the dreaded disease ever came one's way. The day after I was diagnosed with cancer I tried to read the article again, this time through tears. In my disturbed state I was unable to concentrate, so I brought the article with me to the hospital, to read when (as I hoped) I would have recovered some calm.

A day or two after the operation I crawled out of bed and made my way to the oratory in the hospital. I was feeling weak so I just sat inside the door. There was an old man, obviously a patient also, as he was wearing pyjamas and a dressing gown, sitting in a wheelchair in front of the tabernacle. There was no one else in the chapel. The old man looked back, not saying anything, but I got the impression he was calling me. On the second or third occasion when he turned slightly to look back at me I trusted my intuition and went up to him. I got into the seat beside him. We started to talk. He asked me how I came to be there. I told him – cancer. I told him how scared I was, really scared. Then I told him about the article written by Fr Nash and the consolation I got from what the article said each letter of the word 'cancer' stood for: C = Christ; A = Approaching; N = Now. Then I got stuck! I could not recall what the last three letters stood for. The old man knew what they stood for. He pointed his forefinger deliberately and said, 'C = Christ; E = Everlastingly; R = Rewarding.' Astonished, I asked him how on earth he knew this – had he read the article too? He smiled and whispered to me, 'Sure, I am Fr Nash.' I was stunned. We sat together in silence.

When two people feel that death is imminent, I suppose it is natural that they can become very close in a short time. We shared our inner world and feelings as if in some mysterious way we had known each other all our lives. Fr Nash shared with me a confidence I shall always treasure. I told him about my fear of what the future might hold for me – secondaries. He calmed me by pointing out that that was a bridge I could not cross until I came to it. I sensed in the silence that followed that if and when I did come to that bridge, I would be given to know then, and only then, how to cross it safely. For the time being I must simply trust.

Now it was time for us to part and he asked me if I would come to the oratory at the same time tomorrow. I said I could not promise to be there at the exact same time. Fr Nash laughed and said, 'Sure, come to think of it, I'm not sure where I will be this time tomorrow either.' Next day, when I did get the opportunity to look for him, I was told that he had been taken to a nursing home. I never saw him again. Our encounter lasted only a few minutes, but it will stand the test of time, for it was full of truth and compassion.

As I write, Fr Nash is gone to God, but he will always occupy a special place in my heart.

## HOPE

When I was in my late teens I was making my mother's bed one day when I found a note written by her and placed under the mattress. The words touched me deeply and I remember them clearly: 'To hope means hoping when everything seems hopeless; otherwise it is not a virtue at all.'

I sat down quietly for a while to give those words time to become engraved on my heart. Then I carefully placed the note back under the mattress and forgot that I had ever seen it. One can sense when one is treading on holy ground. Little did I know then that twenty-five years later those words would become my lifeline.

When I came home from hospital after the surgery, I would wake up at night and the only thing written on the blackboard of my mind was 'CANCER'. It had arrived on my doorstep. I had 'IT'. I would reflect on the goodness of my husband and the holy innocence of our children, and my heart would feel heavy as lead, about to break. Then when I was almost overwhelmed with grief at the thought of dying, my mother's words would come back to me from the distant past: 'To hope means hoping when everything seems hopeless; otherwise it is not a virtue at all.' I felt hopeless, so this was surely a golden opportunity to practise the virtue of hope. It seemed an insurmountable challenge, a challenge to transcend myself with all my fear. It was as if my mother, now gone to heaven, was reaching me through the medium of those words, and empowering me to 'hold on'. And so eventually I would fall asleep again, feeling hopelessly hopeful.

We have a double swing in our garden on which I love to swing along with the children. There is a sense of timelessness on a swing, which the child in me enjoys to this day. Our youngest child, Paul, then seven years old, got great pleasure from swinging alongside his mum. I was home from hospital only a few days when one morning Paul smiled up into my face and said, 'Mum, come on the swing with me!' I was still in a daze with shock and heartbreak, and here was our youngest asking me to go swinging with him. His innocence was so pure and he so obviously could have no idea of what I was going through that I had not the heart to refuse him. As we swung he was beside himself with joy, while I was beside myself with a grief bordering on despair. We were alongside each other, but we were worlds apart. The child was conscious only of life. I was conscious only of death. I felt so alone and yet so much at one with all those people who were suffering from cancer or any other disease. I knew the child was unable to be with me in my distraught state.

After some time I was touched by an unexpected grace. The child's very innocence revealed that spirit of life – life which transcends death. As the scales began to fall from my eyes, I could see that while the child was unable to be with me in my broken reality, I was being called upon to be with him in his holy reality. I recognised that the road I was travelling on was the Road to Emmaus. Like the two disciples, I had been so preoccupied and heavy with the thoughts of what had happened in the recent past that I was unaware of the 'stranger' in the form of an innocent child. I had gone out to the swing full of fear; I returned to the kitchen to prepare a meal – full of hope.

## LIGHT IN THE NIGHT

For about four years before I was diagnosed as having cancer I felt more comfortable in bed at night if there was a dim light in the hallway. I felt that if I woke during the night, the light would reassure me that I still had my sight, that I could still see. I had always enjoyed perfect sight, so I often wondered why I had this instinctive fear. Without the light I knew that I could wake up during the night with the dreadful sensation of having gone blind.

From the time I was operated on for cancer I never felt the need for this light. Again I wondered why. Then, one day, a doctor said to me: 'You know, Jean, you are really lucky!' In dismay I asked him how he could come to that conclusion as I was still trying to come to terms with the terrifying fact that I had cancer. He explained that the tissue under the nail is a very rare type of tissue in the body, but it is also to be found at the back of the eye. So the malignant melanoma could have struck the tissue behind my eyes just as easily as it had struck that under my thumbnail. 'In other words,' he said, 'you could have suddenly gone blind!' Now I knew why I had felt the need for that light in the night before I had surgery for cancer.

## A CHILD'S GIFT OF DISCERNMENT

Having put the two younger children, Anthony and Paul, to bed and said the night prayers with them, I then went into Teresa's bedroom to do likewise. I was feeling a bit 'down'. Having said the night prayers with Teresa and kissed her goodnight, I thought I had managed to cover up my feelings of 'quiet desperation'. Jim was out visiting a neighbour. Sitting down in the two-seater I was now in a place inwardly that is too sad for tears. Next thing, I heard two little feet scurrying up the hallway! It was Teresa. Running across the floor in her nightie she caught me by my two arms and, shaking me with great intensity, said, 'Mammy, where is your HOPE'? The raw courage and fight-back spirit of her whole countenance was infinitely larger than her eleven-year-old little self. When one log is on fire, another log put beside it can catch fire too. As Teresa put her arms around me it was as if I caught the fire of Teresa's passion for life, her courage and, above all, her strength.

I sometimes wonder if I would be alive today if it were not for the way Teresa empowered me that night not to lose the will to live. I read somewhere that children hear not so much what we adults are saying, but rather what we are not saying. Teresa heard what I was not saying that night as I said the night prayers with her. With fierce fire and fury she fought the good fight for both of us – and won!

## THE IMPOSSIBLE IS POSSIBLE

For some time after the cancer surgery I had to return to the surgeon for a monthly check-up. I suppose when you feel you are drowning, you tend to clutch at any straw. I remember one straw I grasped that turned out to be a nettle – and stung the life out of me! It happened when my surgeon told me that the interval between check-ups could now be lengthened to three months. This stirred a ray of hope in me and I immediately asked: 'As time goes by, does it become less likely to return?' The surgeon looked at me long and thoughtfully, and then said: 'Yes, you can *begin* to forget about it when you are eighty.' I thanked him and managed to leave the room without letting him see me shudder.

My husband and children were waiting eagerly for me when I came out of the doctor's. We had promised to bring the children to the pantomime in which Brendan Grace was starring. So as not to spoil the day for them, I just said I was fine. The pantomime was very enjoyable but inwardly I was in turmoil. I felt annoyed with myself for having asked that stupid question. I was amazed at the surgeon's lack of sensitivity to an obvious cry from the heart. I was hurt and disappointed by his measured response to my question. No doubt my question sprang from an unconscious need – a desperate need to be relieved at least to some extent of the heavy burden that cancer had brought upon me psychologically. I longed to be relieved of some of the weight – even just a little bit!

God knew the yearning in my heart and answered my prayer in a most unusual way – through the medium of Brendan Grace in the pantomime! As part of a hilarious act, Brendan, a man of stout build and large stature, dived in and out through a window on stage in a way that seemed impossible for a man of his size. I reckoned that if Brendan Grace could defy the laws of gravity in such a seemingly impossible way, then so could I. There and then I decided to let the surgeon's words fly in and out through the window of my mind, and not allow myself be weighed down by them. More important still, I was given the grace to begin to let go of that quiet desperation which had prompted the question in the first place.

## THE POWER OF OUR THOUGHTS

A few months later, during a routine medical check-up I asked the surgeon if there was any book I could read that would help me understand the form of cancer I had. He said with fierce conviction in his eyes, 'The less you know about it the better as you have a *deadly* form of cancer.' On hearing this news conveyed in such a heartless way I felt like killing him there and then! Instead, I let silence fall, and in that split second of inner stillness a remarkable thing happened. It was revealed to me that instead of studying the disease itself, it would be far wiser for me to study the self that succumbed to the disease in the first place and in doing so release her with compassion. Standing up I thanked him with a big smile! He looked at me somewhat puzzled. By the time I had reached the door, something in me knew that I was letting myself out of more than one room. I was getting out of the very place in me that had unconsciously made room for the cancer in the first place. Thanks to the surgeon's bedside manner, I woke up!

When I returned home it dawned on me that when I was engrossed in watching a film on TV, I would forget about the cancer. Once the film was over the weight of the word 'cancer' and the dread of dying would return, yet with a difference. It would be diminished somewhat by the break from it. It felt as if there was now some space around the cancer. Then it dawned on me that it wasn't the cancer itself that was weighing me down emotionally. It was my *thoughts* about it. The very thoughts, which appeared to validate my fear, were in reality the cause of it. By simply dropping the thoughts of it, I was dropping my identification with it.

To help me focus on something more creative I began reading books such as *Love, Medicine and Miracles* by Doctor Bernie Siegel and *Gentle Giants* by Penny Brohn (co-founder of the Bristol Cancer Help Centre). These books enabled me to see the cancer in a new light. Above all they encouraged me not to be discouraged by doctors' prognoses! We are blessed to have doctors but we are more blessed to have an inner self that is in union with a knowing that is beyond all intellectual knowledge.

In the meantime I mentioned to Sr Mary that I could not understand how this eminent surgeon could operate on me one day, saving my life, and months later, during a routine check-up, speak to me with a callous look that would kill anyone in the whole of their health! Then I added, as if talking to myself, 'There is something about me that touches a raw nerve in him.' Mary gave me a knowing smile. She then told me that the surgeon's younger brother had suffered from the exact same form of cancer I had, i.e. malignant melanoma of the nail tissue, and he had died shortly after being diagnosed. The surgeon had taken a two-year career break after his brother's death to study the disease in depth. I can only guess that the surgeon felt both sad and angry because he could not save the life of the brother he dearly loved.

## THE WOUNDED CHILD

I still remember a moment that hurt me deeply as a child. I was only five years old at the time. My mother had given me a bunch of roses to bring to the teacher for the school altar. I was thrilled. In the mind of a small child, the distance between our house and the school seemed long. As I got nearer the school my step quickened. My hand holding the roses was hot and my heart was racing with excitement in anticipation of seeing the teacher's face light up when I gave her the flowers. The altar was high up on the classroom wall.

When I arrived the teacher was up on a step-ladder arranging it, so she did not see me coming. But one of the girls in the class – a smartypants – saw me. She somehow managed to grab the roses out of my hand. I can still see her walking up to the teacher with a big smile, saying nothing, but conveying the lie that she had brought the roses. The teacher thanked her for being such a good girl. I sank into my desk. My world had collapsed. I saw myself as a failure because I was unable to hold my own. I felt ashamed because, paralysed as I was by feeling bad and stupid, I could not stand up for myself. I despised Smartypants for what she did, but I despised myself even more for my failure to cope with the situation. I can still see the eager look on my mother's face when I went home that afternoon and she asked me how the teacher had reacted to the flowers. I could not bring myself to tell her the truth about what had happened.

The Wounded Child, the Hurt Child is trapped in everyone's psyche. In other words, there is a little person whose psychological development has not kept pace with the growth of the physical body. It is buried alive in us and can make its presence felt when we react in an exaggerated or disproportionate way in an adult situation. Some are more conscious of their Wounded Child than others. It took cancer to make me aware of my Hurt Child and of how little I had done to heal its own crushed heart. Some adults have painful childhood memories of being put down by an authority figure, say a teacher; being laughed at by their peers; being unduly criticised. The list is endless. The wound in some may be deeper than in others, but the point to remember is that we carry the hurts of childhood into adult life.

About three months after my operation I was at a social gathering one evening. One of those present was talking about something she had read in the newspaper and said with enthusiasm, 'I see that some researchers are on the brink of finding a cure for cancer.' One would expect that I would have been overjoyed at this news; that I would have made it my business to get talking to the person whom I had overheard. But something inside held me back. It was only then that I discovered to my astonishment that there was a part of me that was not interested in being cured. When I got home I reflected on my reaction or, rather, my lack of reaction, to what I had heard. At first I felt frustrated and began to scream inwardly, 'But surely this cannot be true – it does not make sense!' When I calmed down I lovingly confronted that part of me that was lagging behind so lethargically, that part of me that transpired to be the Wounded Child in me. I knew that I must listen to what it had to say. In its anguish it spoke up boldly. The gist of the conversation between myself and my Wounded Child went like this:

*Wounded Child:* In your sophisticated adult world you have no room in your life for me. You are ashamed of me because I am so little, so vulnerable and so wounded. You ignore me. You do not even wish to know me.

*Adult Self:* When did I ignore you? People are always commenting on how joyful I am; how childlike I can be. I laugh so easily – surely that is making room for you in me?

*Wounded Child:* See, you still ignore me. You are talking now to the Healthy Child in you. You do not wish to acknowledge me – the Wounded Child in you. It is so much easier for you to walk along the other side of the road and leave me with my wounded self. A wound left unattended can fester and become malignant. It is I who have cancer. It is I who am tired of living, tired of dying. It is to your detriment that you ignore me!

*Adult Self:* I recognise you now! I remember you now! I recall all the times you wanted to cry but it was never the appropriate time to let you do so. I could not reveal your presence in me because I knew you would be despised. Your tears would be seen as weakness and I would be looked upon as a failure.

*Wounded Child:* Yes, I could see your dilemma! That is why I have tried to bear with you for so long. But now [crying] I cannot contain those tears any longer. Too many have accumulated. I am afraid we are both going to drown!

*Adult Self:* No! I will ensure that you're not destroyed by all that unexpressed sorrow. I regret that your wound had to become malignant for me to put aside my pride and acknowledge you as mine. But the truth is, Wounded Child, you *are* mine. That truth is going to set us both free. In God's own time you will be healed and our joy will be as profound as was your former despair. In my selfless effort to love you into wholeness I shall be healed also. We will be all the richer for having walked through this valley of darkness together.

The exhausted child sleeps in the adult's arms.

One day, while observing the Wounded Child in me, these lines came to mind:

> When they cast their shadows on you
> No need to hide your pain
> But let the sunshine of my love
> Seep through your wound like rain.
>
> Hold fast to this my little one
> Your day of healing has begun
> On you the light of Christ has shone
> For now you know there is only One.

After this insight I felt I was in the process of becoming more whole. I could see cancer as a friend in disguise trying to awaken me to embrace the whole of my reality; to take a positive view of what seemed so negative.

It was only some years later that I discovered that stress can cause the immune system to malfunction, so that disease takes over. Some experts in this field agree that there is a death wish in each one of us even if we are not aware of it.[1] It would seem that 15 to 20 per cent of all cancer patients unconsciously wish to die. They welcome a serious illness as a way to escape their problematic world. About 60 per cent of cancer patients do what is expected of them in order to get well, but in reality the thrust of their whole being is not engaged in the task of getting well. Then there are about 20 per cent who refuse to see themselves as victims of some alien force 'out there', knocking them down at random. They assume responsibility for their lives and set about learning how they may call on their own energies, untapped reserves and healing powers. So they question the doctor to find out what they can do for themselves.

Some weeks after I had had surgery, a friend came to see me. She asked with genuine concern: 'What if IT comes back?' When she had left and was out of earshot I shouted 'F... *IT*! I have had enough of IT!' That person's question woke me up to the fact that my whole being wished to throw its weight behind my effort to become well.

It was only when I began to observe, remember, understand and acknowledge the Wounded Child within me that I began to be healed. It was only when I became conscious of my painful childhood memories, which had been repressed, and when I allowed myself to experience their original emotional

1.  Cf. Bernie Siegel, *Love, Medicine and Miracles*, Arrow Books, 1986.

intensity that my childhood psyche gave way to healing and redemption. It seemed as if the cancer *had* come to light in order for the Wounded Child in me to come to healing. Then I could visualise the cancer starting to die within me. It was as if it began to die of starvation because it only had as much life as I had unconsciously been giving it. I stumbled on to my path to healing when I became conscious of what I was unconsciously doing to myself – disowning the Wounded Child within me.

## WALKING IN A NEW DIRECTION

It is not easy to come to terms with cancer. It was not easy for me. But each day as I went for a walk along the road by our house I felt myself gaining a little more strength – strength to face IT, or rather to face my *fear* of IT.

One day I looked at the green fields and the house and the lovely view from it, as if for the first time. Perhaps it was also as if for the last time. Then it dawned on me that I was looking at it as a stranger passing by. I had not been able to receive all this as pure gift. I was unable to receive. I was not only outside my own house, but was in some sense a stranger to it. It was as if I lived a certain distance from myself, as if I only existed on the surface of life. This realisation filled me with great sadness. Indeed, it occurred to me that it would not be a big deal for me to die now, because in a sense I was already 90 per cent lifeless. I stayed with this pain, letting myself feel its weight. It seemed like the weight of my own corpse. Paradoxically, as I did so, I began to sense the littleness and the greatness of the life that was still in me. More important still, I began to sense its potential to swallow up my lifelessness in victory. The victim had it in her to become the victor, by simply changing her focus, that is, by paying more attention to the life still in her, rather than to the cancer.

As I turned for home my step became brisker, my head a little higher and my shoulders a little less drooped. I began to feel a new energy in me that awakened courage from her slumber. This courage would enable me to face and experience pain, especially emotional pain; it would enable me to face fear and redeem with compassion that helpless Wounded Child in me. I knew that if I were to live, I must make all this my own, in my own time.

On my return home I went intuitively into each room in the house. It struck me for the first time that all of them were painted the same colour – primrose yellow! Even the sheets on the beds were primrose yellow. Although I didn't know anything about the significance of colour, one thing was clear: I was stuck on yellow! I sat down and, letting my imagination go, I began to picture each room painted a different colour – marshmallow pink, pale lilac, soft green. The carpets in the bedrooms were well worn by now, so clearly we needed new carpets! These would be in a deeper shade than the subtle colour on the walls and would set the house ablaze. The only snag was money! We simply could not afford it, however desirable it might be.

By the time my husband came in from work I was not seeing straight. All I could see was every colour in the rainbow and every room in its own distinctive shade. Jim listened with some amusement and a lot of tolerance! Shortly afterwards, through an unexpected bequest, the money needed to do the job came to us. I was able to redecorate the house and buy little desks for the children so that they could do their homework at their own desk on coming in from school in the evening. It took about two months to complete all this, and at the end, while I was pleased, I also knew there was an element of despair in the work. I now felt that even if I did have to die soon I had created the best possible living conditions for my husband and children to go on with their lives without my being around.

When the painting and decorating was complete, I just loved the new colours. They seemed to symbolise the new life I was trying to embrace. Later on, I was talking to a friend one day who has great insight into the workings of the human heart. I asked her if she could make any sense of my wanting to repaint the house as a way of overcoming cancer. She explained that, in fact, I was following a sure instinct. Colour is life and she said, 'It is obvious that you are opening up to *new* life.' That explanation rang true for me.

## A FRIEND DIES

About eight months after my surgery, a friend died from cancer. She had a devoted husband and a very young family. Some months before her death she telephoned me. I can still recall her voice on the phone trying to give me encouragement by saying, 'Jean, THINK POSITIVE!' At that time she was going through a difficult period having treatment for secondaries. I appreciated the effort she made to comfort me and inspire me with hope, but when I put down the phone I wept for both of us. When the person who comes to comfort and console you is herself in a pathetic state, which she tries to transcend in order to help you, you can glimpse a spark of the divine.

Shortly before her death she invited a few of her friends to Mass in her house. Most of those present had had surgery for cancer. There was great empathy in the group. The peace was palpable. When Mass was over our friend asked us to join hands around the little table which had served as an altar and to join with her in singing 'Jesus, Remember Me'. That evening the word 'remember' came alive for me, took on a new meaning: 'Jesus, put me together again when you come into your Kingdom.' Our friend was in touch with her brokenness, and she was also in touch with the One who would remember her – the One who had promised: 'This day you will be with me in Paradise.' It was only then that I discovered the difference between being cured and being healed. One person may be cured of a serious illness by modern medication but not have found inner peace; another person may die from a serious illness but be healed inwardly and die in peace.

When she died I felt very downhearted and confused. I felt angry with God and gave him a piece of my mind! I told him that our friend's death just did not make sense. I could not find any meaning in her death, nor could I understand her dying so young. Needless to say, underneath all this search for meaning and this groping for understanding was my own fear that the Lord would make a similar mistake by taking me. I was trying to get the message across to him not to make any more mistakes! But the Lord was patient with me, for he is full of gentleness and compassion, and he understood my anxiety and my grief.

Every storm eventually blows itself out and so too did my anger with God. Those words of the saints came to my mind: to possess him who cannot be understood is to renounce all that can be understood. Then one day he lovingly revealed to me the root of all my troubles. I recognised the voice of the Wounded Lover: 'You are able to entrust me with your life but you are afraid to entrust me with your death. I am the Lord of both Life *and* Death.' That day I was called to experience a depth of faith in the Risen Lord, a depth of which I had never dreamed.

A priest giving a seminar on coping with bereavement put it beautifully. He said that at birth we emerge from life in the womb into the womb of life; at death we emerge from the womb of life into the fullness of life. Then he added these lines:

> Death breaks an earthly tie
> but love survives when grief has passed,
> for love can never die.

Our friend is now in Paradise and I am at peace.

## A RETREAT

Twelve months after my surgery for cancer I became aware of my need for emotional and spiritual healing. So I took myself off to a Cistercian monastery for a four-day retreat. I went there to reflect and pray, and, hopefully, with the help and guidance of one of the monks, to untie the emotional knot that had its origins in the Wounded Child in me.

I had some happy childhood memories of my mother hiring a car occasionally to bring the whole family to the monastery. Later I had often stayed there as a guest for several days and loved to fall in with the Cistercian way of life – their rhythm of work and prayer, and being present daily at Mass and at the Morning and Evening Prayer of the monks. The only thing I never did appreciate was being woken at 4.00 a.m. by the great church bell calling the monks to the first office of the day!

My four-day retreat began on a Monday morning, bright and early. Those four days will always stand out as a turning-point on my inward journey. First of all, by chance or divine coincidence I met a nun who was on retreat there. After we had talked for a while she offered me some tapes to listen to on the theme of The Healing Journey. As I listened to those tapes I felt like someone in the middle of a desert, dying of thirst, being offered sparkling cool water from a mountain stream. It was as if life itself was reaching me with its healing touch through the medium of those tapes. The whole atmosphere of the place was quietly on fire with God and I never felt more in need of him.

I enjoyed those days but the fourth day was coming fast and I still did not feel ready to talk to a monk. However, taking my courage in my hands, I made an appointment to see one of the community, not knowing what I was going to say. Walking under the shade of the great trees I prayed that the monk would be inspired to give me the life-giving word. My prayer was answered.

As I talked with the monk I began to see that everyone's journey in life is made up of sorrowful mysteries and joyful mysteries. I was now being brought to see that life is a mystery to be lived rather than a problem to be solved. The monk did not erase my pain but rather showed me how to walk with it; how to be patient with all that was unsolved in my heart; to try to love the questions and not to seek the answers which could not be given until I was ready to live them. The point was for me to *live* everything. I must live the questions now and gradually, without my even noticing it, I would one day live into the answers. I came to realise that my story was a unique version of the story of everyone who ever walked this earth – and so it was the story of God himself. I no longer felt isolated. I felt connected to all humankind, and to God. I discovered that it is only in so far as we can embrace the Good Friday in our lives that we can experience the Easter Sunday.

As I strolled once again under the shade of those trees I no longer felt like a caterpillar weighed down and worn out from struggling. Now my spirit soared peacefully above the trees like a butterfly. Instead of fighting the sorrow that is inevitable in life I entered into the mystery of it. It began to yield its hidden beauty to me and this had a fragrance all its own.

## SECONDARIES

At the end of my four days in the monastery I knelt in the Abbey church and prayed. The tears flowed freely. They were tears of joy and relief, but they were also tears of sorrow, because I somehow knew, even though I had no visible signs, that I already had secondaries. I had had my routine medical check-up and everything seemed fine. Yet as I knelt there in the Abbey church I was alone with the knowledge that I would have to face another operation and God knows how much more suffering. At the same time, however, I was leaving the monastery conscious not only of my secondaries, but also of the abundant *new* life awakened in me.

About a month later I went to a healing workshop in Dublin as I was not feeling very well, though medical tests did not tally with my hunch that I had secondaries. I did not fully understand the significance of the healing I would experience while there. At this workshop I met a nun named Sr Anne. After chatting for some time I shared with her my dread of secondaries. She was most understanding and tried to reassure me. Yet, deep down, I felt like someone standing in the middle of the ocean trying to stop the tide from coming in. Later when we were having a coffee break I could not contain the 'inner knowing' that I had secondaries and again said to the nun, 'Oh God! I can't leave the poor little children – what will I do?' Once more Sr Anne was most kind to me and again tried to reassure me. The next day, I happened to be passing by while Sr Anne was getting something out of a press. Turning around I heard myself cry out, 'What will I do?' Something snapped in Sr Anne and she shouted, 'LET IT!' Suddenly I felt like a frightened five-year-old child clinging to her life the way she would cling to a sweet with her clenched fist! Sr Anne's unexpected reaction knocked the sweet out of my hand. Now my hands and fingers were wide open, letting life flow in and out *through* them. It was as if I was free-falling, clinging to *nothing* any more, not even my life! While free-falling I suddenly realised, at a level deeper than words, that death is not the opposite of life; that death is the opposite of birth. In that moment I discovered the ground of my being – the 'I AM' that was never born and would never die. As I surrendered I could feel every cell in my body relaxing – thanks to Sr

Anne's patience and *impatience* with me! This revelation was so subtle, it would take years for me to fully understand its impact on me, much less be able to put it into words. Then one day the first three lines in *A Course in Miracles* came alive for me:

> Nothing real can be threatened
> Nothing unreal exists
> Herein lies the peace of God.

At that workshop I also met Sr Bernadette. She told me, 'People say I have something [healing power] in my hands. I don't know!' She was so relaxed and laughed so easily, I had a hunch that people might be right. However, we did not exchange addresses or telephone numbers, and after the weekend we went our separate ways, not expecting to meet again.

About two months later (which was about fifteen months after my first operation), I was going about the house doing my usual chores one Friday morning, when I felt a lump under my left armpit. It felt like a floating golf ball! I was alone. My husband was out and the children were gone to school. I managed to get a message to Jim to come home. I tried to hold back the ocean of tears that I was too frightened to shed until my husband arrived. I felt that my spirit was healed but wondered was it too late for the Good News to reach my poor earthly body, living as we do on different levels simultaneously. When my husband opened the door I ran to him and, throwing myself into his arms, I sobbed my heart out, crying, 'I don't want to die, I don't want to die!' He hugged me, tried to reassure me and was a tower of strength.

## MORE SURGERY

We managed to make an appointment to see my surgeon some hours later. I went with my bag packed ready to go straight into hospital. The surgeon examined me lying flat on my back and then said he could find nothing of any significance! I felt frustrated because I knew the 'golf ball' slipped away when I lay down on my back. It was only when I was sitting upright that one could feel it. I was quite sure I was not imagining it. In my distraught state I mentioned that I could find it only when sitting upright, but by now he was sure that there was nothing significant there. The result was that we left the doctor's office with mixed feelings, torn between a vague sense of relief and a keen sense of apprehension. In my ears were his words that I should come back for my routine check-up in one month's time. That day must have been the longest I ever lived!

Next morning, Saturday, I woke early and again knew that I was in real trouble. I felt I had caused my husband enough anguish, so without saying anything to him I slipped out and went to my family doctor. This time I took the initiative by asking him to let me find the floating 'golf ball' myself. Sitting in an upright position, and leaning forward a little, I found the lump. Then he examined it and was so alarmed that he phoned the surgeon on the spot. But it was Saturday and the surgeon was away. It was only hours later that the doctor made contact with him. And when he did, he was told that the examination the previous day had shown nothing and I could come back in a week if I was still worried.

As I felt that my life was at stake I thought it would be unwise to wait for a week. My husband and I returned on Monday morning. This time the surgeon found the floating 'golf ball' and told me gravely that it was an enlarged lymph gland. They would remove it, but that did not mean it was malignant. This gave me a ray of hope and I entered hospital straightaway.

I went into hospital with very mixed feelings. I had known intuitively for about three months that I had secondaries, but I had been hoping my intuition was wrong. I was glad because I knew I would now have the medical attention I needed. I was sad for my husband and children, and I was fearful of what lay before me.

As the various tests were carried out on me, I could sense that things were bad. For one thing, my blood count was very low. I found it difficult to sleep that night, as my pulse rate was far too high – out of sheer panic no doubt! This caused a throbbing in my head, and when I asked the nurse about this she said that in fact it was due simply to fright. I remained in this state until I went down to theatre.

Before I knew it, it was four o'clock the next morning and the surgery was over. The minute I woke up I knew that the lump was malignant. Yet with this dreadful realisation came the grace to accept it. My pulse rate slowed to normal and my panic gave way to peace.

When my husband came in to visit me later that day he told me how restless he had been during the night, unable to sleep, clinging to the hope that the gland was not malignant. Then he said: 'I woke up at 4.00 a.m. and I knew it was malignant, but a strange thing happened. I accepted it and became quite peaceful and went back to sleep.' A coincidence? Perhaps, but I believe that such empathy between a husband and wife is not unusual, especially when going through such a crisis. He brought me a Walkman with some of my favourite tapes, including those of the Jesuit, Tony de Mello, on Peace, Love, Joy, and the music of Phil Coulter, particularly his 'Serenity'.

My surgeon told me he had removed the swollen gland and one on either side of it, and had done a biopsy on the other glands in the area, and he was waiting for the result. I gathered that the swollen gland was in fact malignant. Again, I was told that radium treatment or chemotherapy 'would be of dubious value' in my case. You can imagine how pleased I was when he came in to tell me that in fact none of the other glands were affected. He remarked that he was 'very pleased' with this result, and so, needless to say, was I!

I remember asking the surgeon one day, 'If the cancer comes back again, where is it likely to strike?' He was standing at the end of the bed at the time and he threw his hands up in the air and said simply, 'Oh, ANYWHERE!' He then left the ward, having no idea of the inner devastation his answer caused me. I knew that if I gave in to my feelings I would start crying and not be able to stop, so I went to the phone to ask a priest friend to offer Mass for me.

Coming back to bed, I was aware that the other three women in the ward with me had heard the conversation and had a pretty good idea of how it had hit me. So I jokingly said, 'Girls, something tells me I had better make for my fall-out shelter.' They knew what I meant. I put on my earphones and settled down to listen to the music of Coulter, and the wisdom of de Mello.

Through the medium of Phil Coulter's music I felt connected to a healing energy beyond human comprehension, an energy that I have no doubt is divine. I stayed with this healing energy, flowing through the medium of Phil Coulter's music and de Mello's spirituality, and I found that I was full of peace and was able to laugh again.

That same day another surgeon, known to me as he had operated on one of our children for tonsils, came into the ward and recognised me. He came over and asked me what I was doing there. I told him in one word – cancer. His words of hope and consolation were charged with so much empathy and compassion. Healing emanated from his whole countenance, and I was very much the better of his coming.

There is always, of course, a humorous side to hospital life and the company helps so much to cheer one up. I became close to the other three women in the ward and we shared our fears and pains, our hopes for better health and the stories of our families. One of the women gave me a book to read and it was just what I needed at that time. The loving providence of God works in our lives through the goodness and kindness of others.

Before I left the hospital I knew I would have to bring up again the question about the likelihood of the return of the cancer. In answer to my queries, the surgeon told me of patients on whom he had operated ten and fifteen years before, and who were still alive and well. These words were a real boost to my morale and confidence. And I found myself saying, with Julian of Norwich, all shall be well, and all shall be well, and all manner of things shall be well.

A month later, when I returned for my routine check-up, the surgeon said to me, 'Wasn't it great that you had the good sense to come back that time?' Smiling, I said, 'Yes, especially when I heard what I wanted to hear.' The most important thing was that there was no time lost, and both doctor and patient were glad about that. All's well that ends well!

The strange thing is that it was only after being operated on for secondaries that I had a subtle feeling deep down that I had left cancer behind me. I knew that there was no logic to this hunch. Then on my next routine medical check-up with my surgeon I sounded him out! He told me that there were two schools of thought with regard to the rare form of cancer I had. He said that if I had been operated on in America that the lymph glad under my left armpit would have been removed at the same time as they removed the first joint of my left thumb. But he said, 'In this part of the world we prefer to let any remaining cancerous cells in the system gather in the lymph gland *first* and *then* remove it.' I told the surgeon that I was glad I was living in this part of the world as the approach here made more sense to me! Now I did not see the malignant lymph gland as an enemy but rather as a friend that was willing to sacrifice its own life in order to save me. The body has an intelligence of its own, and when we listen to it and honour it, miracles happen.

## CONVALESCING

My days in hospital were coming to an end and it was time for me to return home. While being glad that the operation was successfully over, I was physically weak. I did not feel up to housework and looking after young children straightaway. I needed time to be alone with myself to integrate the trauma of the last ten days.

It happened that my friend, Sr Mary, had ten days' leave from duty and intended making a private retreat. My friendship with Mary and her religious sisters goes back to my childhood and schooldays. She invited me to her convent where she would spend her ten days taking care of me while I convalesced. This was surely an offer I couldn't refuse! Mary persuaded me that she would enjoy spending her retreat days this way. When I told my husband, he was delighted for me and grateful to

Mary. Looking back now I can see that those ten days' convalescence were heaven-sent to save my life.

After surgery for cancer many patients are told, 'Go home and live life exactly as you have been living it up to now.' Being in a state of shock, many patients are likely to do just that. Common sense told me to do otherwise: to stop and look at the direction in which I was going, to listen to my inmost self. I began to ask myself questions, such as: 'What is cancer trying to tell me about myself, my relationships, my attitudes to life and everything in it?' It was obvious that there was something wrong and that I had better set it right before it was too late. Slowly but surely it dawned on me that I could do this by simply changing my way of *seeing* life.

I could see that cancer was trying to reveal to me an accumulation of 'swallowed tears'. Tears I had not wept because it never seemed the appropriate time to weep them. All the suffering I had swallowed had got stuck, jammed up inside me and I could no longer contain it. When the dam collapsed, the flood manifested itself in the form of cancer.

During those ten days I arranged to meet a priest counsellor. I talked to him about how much I looked forward to going home, but how I dreaded the thought of my first day there when my husband would have gone out to work and the children to school. I would be alone at the kitchen sink, 'broken'. These words welled up from gut level. My deepest self was talking. 'Broken.' I knew I was broken. The silence which followed was sacred, because I was now fully experiencing in the depths of myself my Wounded Child. Then I began to cry. It was as if a dam holding back an enormous flood had suddenly collapsed. The tears flowed like the Niagara Falls. I knew this priest could handle the situation and bring me through it safely. The time was ripe to let go – to let my heart break. The counsellor did indeed handle the outburst beautifully and when I had finished crying he told me that I had cried tears that needed to be shed for over forty years. I knew he was right. This meeting was painful but it was therapeutic at a profound level. Later, while at Mass, those words, 'He BROKE the bread', came alive for me.

We met once more during the ten days. Now I could think straight. He showed me, with great gentleness, how to take responsibility for my life and everything in it. He enabled me to draw on my own power to give birth to my *real* self. A great healing process was set in motion when I began to make conscious contact with my own creative centre and get a sense of my real self. It was only then it began to dawn on me that there was more to cancer than the physical aspect of it, that the physical can be a symptom of the psychological. I no longer felt a victim of this strange and terrible disease 'out there'. I owned IT. I was on safe ground, the ground of my own being, the ground given to me as a gift from God. The priest also suggested that I light a candle each morning and sit before it prayerfully, if only for a few minutes. After trying this for some time I found it more helpful to place a crucifix in front of the lighted candle. I would then sit in silence, and looking at the cross I would breathe out the cancer, and looking at the lighted candle I would breathe in the light, which was the risen life. I found this way of meditation a tremendous help. Before we parted I asked the priest one last question: 'How can I be sure it is God's will for me to live?' He explained to me that life is a gift and that 'God in you is willing you to live'.

In a sense I doubt if I ever worked as hard in my whole life as I did during those ten days. By releasing my stored-up energies I summoned up my own buried energies for inner healing. It was re-creative work. I was co-operating with God to re-create myself *from within*. I discovered that faith can move mountains because I had seen mountains falling in my psyche. Only Mary knew the powerful work that was going on behind the seeming passivity. I suspect that some of the sisters felt I might go 'nutty' in a room on my own, without even a radio. One day Mary brought me a radio and we both laughed because we both knew that I had no time to listen to it! I shared the joke with the priest counsellor, who replied seriously: 'They need not fear – you only withdraw in order to explore.'

A neighbouring priest who knew about my illness had had my name called out at Knock Shrine, Co. Mayo, for prayers during the Vigil there on the night after my operation. There were ten thousand people walking in procession with lighted candles who heard that request for prayers and who prayed for me. I was deeply touched by this. The power of prayer is beyond all else. At my husband's request, this priest visited me in the convent, and before he left he prayed with me. That night I had this experience:

I woke up about 3.00 a.m., and felt that while I knew I was awake and in possession of my senses, I was as a babe safe in Our Lady's arms. It was as if I had just been born and Our Lady was my mother. I somehow 'knew' that the experience was authentic and next day I shared it with my friend Mary. She simply remarked: 'Don't you remember that priest gave you Our Lady's blessing before he left?'

During those ten days, Mary looked after me with love and care. She brought my meals to my room and took me out for walks when I was able to go. If a friend is someone in whose company you can talk to yourself out loud, then she was that friend. She was able to bear with me no matter what my mood and our shared laughter was such a help.

One day about this time our parish priest made a routine visit to the school where my daughter Teresa was then in class. She told him about Mammy being sick and so next day he kindly came along to visit me. He remarked that he thought the child did not realise the gravity of my condition. But I know Teresa. Her great spirit of hope would come shining through her whole countenance. Her faith would be greater than her fear. Then he said to me: 'And you look so content,' as though to imply that he thought I did not realise the gravity of my condition either! (It was only afterwards that I thought of the words of St Paul about learning to be content in whatever state he was.) He told me about one or two people whom he knew who had had secondaries about eight years previously and they were still alive and well, without any recurrence. When you have been operated on for cancer you love to hear of people who have also had the disease and have survived. We all hear of people who died of cancer, but there have always been survivors and I wanted to identify with them. The conversation was not all serious, and the laughter and good humour he brought to me were therapeutic too.

My husband came to see me during this time, although I had assured him that he would have enough to do with his work and the children. Being unsure about whether or not he would be able to come, he wrote me a long letter, telling me how he felt about the situation, and this letter is one of my treasures to this day.

The sisters were sensitive in their care for me and always seemed to be there when I most needed them. The day I left the convent to return home, I thanked the sisters in their chapel before Mass. My farewell went something like this: 'Dear Friends, this Mass will be offered in thanksgiving for all your kindness to me. I came here ten days ago feeling as though I had been torn apart, having been operated on for cancer twice in the one year, as you might say. I felt shattered by the experience. Tradition tells us that Our Lady *stood* at the foot of the Cross during the Crucifixion. She did not collapse or fall asunder. She did not allow her sorrow to degenerate into sadness. In other words, she never gave in to despair. That image of Our Lady has always been dear to me. During the past ten days you have stood at the foot of my Cross by helping me at every level of my being: physical, emotional and psychological, but above all you have helped me spiritually. I am going home with more life in me now than I have ever known, with a marvellous will to live. God is in me, willing me to live. So instead of being impoverished by cancer, I am being enriched by it. Indeed, if it were not for this illness I would not have come to realise how rich the quality of my life can be, so full of potential for growth in Christ through my brokenness and weakness. When I return home today to my husband and children I know I can count on you to continue remembering me in your prayers. My gratitude is beyond words …'

## TALK ABOUT IT

I had an uncle, my father's only brother, who lived until he was nearly ninety. His spirit remained youthful right to the end of his days. His sense of humour and innate wisdom endeared him to many. I was close to him and he often talked to me about things that he had learned the hard way as he journeyed through life. He shared one lesson in particular with me and I sometimes wonder if I would be alive today if I had not applied it to my own situation. He said to me: 'If you have a problem – put it out there. In other words, TALK ABOUT IT! If you tell enough people, there is sure to be someone who can and will help. If not, there is sure to be someone who knows someone who can and will help!' Obviously one has to be prudent about confiding in people but it is a fact that so often we are not helped because no one knows we need help!

While I was in hospital with cancer, the people of our local community were a tower of strength to me and to my husband and children. They prayed for me night and day, and they helped in every way they could. Some recited the Rosary in our little church each morning. Others prayed at Knock Shrine. Others helped my husband and children in practical ways in the house.

A friend told me of an unusual experience she had had. She could not sleep the night after my operation for secondaries. She had so much empathy with me that she felt as if she herself were going through the trauma. Even when she got up the next morning and was going about the house doing her chores, 'the weight of it all was still upon me'. Then, she said, at around lunchtime 'the weight was lifted off my shoulders with an assurance from an inner voice that there was no need to carry it further.' I was able to tell her that I intuitively knew that her experience was authentic because I remember lying in bed after my operation thinking, 'There must be people out there sharing this burden with me, otherwise I could not possibly feel so free!' The burden was heavy but so many people helped me on the way that I did not feel the weight of it.

It was only then I began to experience what is meant by community and to realise that we are all part of the Mystical Body of Christ. And this did not end when I came home from the hospital. One Sunday morning as I was going in to Mass in our local church I was stopped by an elderly woman. I have already mentioned that a priest had suggested to me that I should pray before a lighted candle each morning. I had planned to buy some candles that weekend. The woman opened her handbag and took out a Lourdes candle. She offered it to me, saying with great conviction: 'Now you must light this candle every morning and pray before it, and you will be well.' I took the candle and she continued, 'Like you, I too was operated on for cancer twice, but I lit my candle each morning and prayed before it and I got well. That was thirty years ago.' I thanked her and during Mass I thanked God for her and for her gift of a candle.

It is widely known that a woman can talk to a woman in a way that she cannot talk to a man. There is a special empathy there. They understand each other precisely because they are both women. To have a woman friend in whom you can confide is a great blessing. As the Bible says: 'A faithful friend is a source of strength; whoever finds one has found a treasure' (Sirach 6:14). I have such a friend in Deirdre. We have been life-long friends. Life is real and pain is unavoidable in this broken world. But when necessary we can communicate our pain to each other and so let go of it. We facilitate each other in our efforts to become more real and therefore more loving persons.

## TELLING DAD

It was not until after my operation for secondaries that I told my father, then almost ninety years old, about the cancer. I gave it a lot of thought before doing so, but decided that I should tell him for two reasons. I felt desperate, and he was my father, with a tremendous spirit of courage and great faith. He had survived hardship and sorrow in his own life, which would have destroyed many another person. He was a survivor. He had been born on a farm in the west of Ireland and his mother died when he was only seven years old. She died on the birth of my father's only brother. His father married again, this time a young widow with six children of her own. Just about seven years later he died, and so at the age of fifteen my father was left homeless. Cast on the waves of the world, he learned how to ride them and how to weather the storms.

He lived out his life to the full, transforming and transcending every obstacle that came his way. He had a great love for the Rosary and recited it faithfully every day of his life. He also had great devotion to St Thérèse of Lisieux. This devotion was not one-sided as she granted him many favours all through his life. Indeed, one night some years ago, St Thérèse came to me in a dream with a message my father wished to convey to me in secret. The memory of that still fills me with wonder and awe.

The second reason I told my Father about the cancer is that I am convinced we ought to share our sorrows as well as our joys with those closest to us, no matter how old they are, otherwise we deprive them of their humanity. I am talking, of course, about elderly people who are capable of understanding and who are not senile. My father was glad I told him and thanked me again and again for sharing with him. He promised to pray for me and I have no doubt that Our Lady and St Thérèse were both given the task of rescuing me!

Sometime later, my father said to me with a conviction that only those with an indomitable spirit and faith such as he had could convey: 'You can forget about the cancer, Jean, it will never come back again.' He was so solemn and so full of peace as he spoke that I believed him. This sharing had brought us closer than ever. It was as if we had somehow been through something formidable together and with the help of God had made it.

During my childhood years Dad had given me many life-giving memories. They go way back to when I was only about three years old. I used chuckle with laughter when he would suddenly sweep me off my feet – up onto his shoulders to give me a 'piggy-back' round the kitchen! His pet name for me was the Blub! At other times he would take me on his lap and sing little songs to me. Now, in his ninetieth year, he asked me one night to sing him to sleep. I was amazed how all his songs of bygone days came back to me. Quiet tears of joy ran down his face as I sang to him and he fell asleep full of peace.

As I write, my Dad is gone to God, so now we are closer than ever.

## TO LIVE IS TO BE SLOWLY BORN

Before I got cancer my general behaviour was coloured by a deep feeling that I owed an apology to the world for my very existence! I can now see all life as a gift and see myself as part of that gift. I have become more assertive now with a much greater sense of my own worth. I now realise that we only know courage to the extent that we know fear. For what is courage if it is not fear transcended? I am no longer afraid to stand my ground and lovingly confront those close to me when necessary. I take time off for recreation and do not feel apologetic about meeting this need in myself. Indeed, this has led to greater understanding and acceptance all round. In a sense, it took cancer to wake me up to stand on my own two feet or, if you like, to make me grow up.

Through prayer and reflection cancer taught me many lessons. Perhaps the most telling lesson of all was a realisation of the importance of giving expression to my negative feelings as quickly as possible once they arise – be they anger, sorrow, grief, fear or any other negative emotion. I came to realise the importance of not waiting until the next day for the appropriate time to give expression to them. By then I may have forgotten them, but they will not have forgotten me. They will have become lodged in me, buried alive. 'Unresolved issues manifest in our tissues.' The buried past does not pass away until we come to terms with it. While it is important that we do not live in the past, it is equally important that we honour memory and face the truth of experiences, which cause us unease so that we can dwell fully in the present with ease. Tears, which are crying out to be wept today, may not be accessible at the appropriate time tomorrow. It came to me that as long as the emotions were blocked there was no way that I could become fully alive. Instead of denying our brokenness, ignoring it or getting mad at it, we are to take it to ourselves and be kind to it. By so doing it will be the means of growth. 'Where there is resentment or holding on to hurts there is a need to forgive the other *in order to free oneself*.' In this broken world it is sometimes necessary to honour our Spirit by walking away and in so doing discover the road to self-realisation. I was brought up to believe that a '*good Christian*' always 'turns the other cheek'. It would take years for me to discover that 'turn the other cheek' is perhaps the most misunderstood statement in the Bible. A deeper understanding reveals an inner surrender to the way things are while outwardly taking necessary action. The important point is to take that action while 'leaving one's heart at the lotus feet of the Lord'. With this newfound awareness I now had access to an inner strength from which I was cut off since childhood. That energy was no longer blocked in me but now flowing. I discovered that a 'no' is as loving as a 'yes' when it arises out of integrity. In listening to our heart we honour our journey of mystery.

It is common knowledge now that in our relationships we cannot express our love for each other until we have first expressed and let go of our anger towards ourselves and each other. I was brought up to believe it was wrong even to *feel* anger, let alone express it! I now see the folly of trying to live in that artificial way. Experience has taught me that anger is a powerful, life-giving force when expressed in a constructive way. It clears the way for love to flow.

I am now living out of my newfound strength with, I trust, great gentleness – for there is nothing more gentle than *real* strength. When we have the courage to feel the truth of our childhood pain and to mourn it, we also mature into mourning the pain we have unintentionally caused other people. We all suffer. We all unknowingly cause suffering. But the Good News is: 'God's Judgement is Compassion'. To put my arms around the whole of myself sounds selfish but it is the most selfless act one can perform. Why? Because in doing so I'm putting my arms around everyone in me – with compassion.

Life is an inward journey. We never arrive. Yet in a sense we are forever arriving. No doubt each day will continue to bring its own challenge for me to face. It is not a case of being home and dry and living happily ever after. The perfection to which we are called is not the perfection of the Pharisee who never makes a mistake, but the perfection that is born of understanding and acceptance – not only of others but also of ourselves. This paves the way for a transformation that can be likened to that part of night, which having reached its darkest hour, gives way to dawn. 'To live is to be slowly born.'

## SR BERNADETTE

About nine months after I had surgery for secondaries, Sr Mary invited me to come with her and eight other sisters for a week to their holiday home by the sea. A priest was coming from England to give a directed retreat to the sisters and I was welcome to join them. The priest, whom I will call Fr Peter, was reputed to be an excellent spiritual director. This proved to be the case, and once more I happened to meet the right person at the right time. I relished every moment of that week, as I walked along the seashore reflecting on my situation and experiences. I was trying to synchronise the discord and the harmony in my life, inevitable in any life worth living. I needed time to do this, and I was helped by the place and the people. The company of the sisters, the guidance of Fr Peter, the power of the sea breaking on the rocks, the sunshine and the wind – all were healing. I was free from all my ordinary duties as housewife and mother. I could see that this week was a gift from God, a time for me to reflect and to remember – put back together – all of me and by the grace of God accept all of me, and with his help look with compassion on all of me. So simple! So difficult!

To cross the threshold from self-judgement and self-accusation to self-acceptance and redemption is not an easy journey. But oh! What ease when we forgive – let go – the disease it has caused us!

My week by the sea was coming to an end, and the evening before I was due to return home I went for a walk down by the shore. I was alone and was listening to 'South Pacific' on my Walkman when an inner voice told me to turn it off. I have learned from experience to recognise and obey this inner movement, so I switched off the cassette player. Suddenly I felt at one with the whole universe and I could feel, as it were, the rug being pulled out from under the whole Cosmos in one gigantic redemptive act. It was like a depth experience of the Paschal Mystery. If I were coming from a different religious background, say Buddhism, I would perhaps express my experience in a different way, as what I'm trying to convey here is beyond words. I had never had such a peak experience of awareness in my whole life. This state lasted some minutes, perhaps, and then I recognised someone walking along the road ahead of me. It was Sr Bernadette, whom I had not seen since the weekend workshop in Dublin months earlier. She was with another nun, and I wondered if she would remember me. She recognised me immediately and we both laughed with joy. The other sister excused herself and left us alone and we talked for about an hour. I told her I had had surgery for secondaries since our last meeting, and she told me that she had discovered in the meantime that she had the gift of healing. She explained to me that her gift was to *communicate the healing power of the Mass* to the person in need of healing. That very morning she was prompted to go back to a second Mass (something she had never felt the urge to do before) as she was going to meet someone that day in need of healing. Her hands become very warm when she is about to meet someone in need of healing and that morning her hands were on fire! As it was now late evening (about 8.30 p.m.) she had been wondering all day who the healing energy was for. Just before meeting me she had said to her companion: 'Well, wouldn't this baffle you! The day is nearly over and I haven't met anyone and my hands are still on fire!' Little wonder then, that as I walked along the road behind her, I picked up the message to switch off the Walkman so as to experience a redemptive power beyond description. I felt a healing energy being released in me, awakening a deep sense of inner freedom.

By the time I got back to the house the sisters were getting anxious as to my whereabouts. Next day I shared the experience with Fr Peter and Sr Mary. That week by the sea will always stand out in my memory as one of the highlights of my entire life.

When I returned home to my family, Sr Bernadette continued to be very supportive. She always seemed to ring me at the right time – when I was assailed by fear of the cancer coming back again. She was able to pick up on my thoughts and feelings. I recall one night in particular when I was depressed with fear of the Big C and had gone to bed. The phone rang at 10 p.m. It was Sr Bernadette. The first question she asked me was 'Jean, where is your trust?' I felt ashamed that she should know that I was such a weakling, but I was glad that she was with me in my weakness. She communicated great faith to me that night and I went back to bed and fell asleep full of peace and confidence in God. Another night she rang to say: 'You are cured.' I was not able to say anything – I was speechless with joy at this assertion. There was silence and then she said: 'I know by the energy in the *tips* of my fingers.' I was still silent. She knew, and the great gentleness, simplicity and *truth* in her voice reached me. Within days of that phone call all fear of cancer had left me, never to return.

## THE OTHERNESS OF THE OTHER

While I was in hospital for my last check-up I was sharing a room with another woman. We were about the same age, both married with young families. She had had surgery for cancer some weeks previously. She was a quiet, reserved type of person and did not wish to speak much about her illness. I respected this. She would say to me: 'Can you imagine how *hurt* my husband and children must be?' Then she would fill up and cry. After a little time I picked what I thought was the right moment to offer her a book that I had found helpful, but she showed no interest. Later on I offered her an audiotape that I thought suitable for someone in her distressed and bewildered condition, but again she declined.

She told me later that when she returned home she did not intend telling her neighbours or friends that she had cancer. She would prefer if they did not know. I assured her that I could understand her feelings, but I also told her how therapeutic I had found it to tell people. I said that I had a great belief in the goodness that is at the heart of everyone and in the power of their prayer. I could see from her doubting smile that she did not share my point of view. I fell asleep that night feeling sad because I was not able to help her help herself.

Next morning I was surprised to see her contentedly sewing buttons on to baby garments, which she had got from the occupational therapist in the hospital. I saw great beauty in this. The baby clothes symbolised new life. She was tending to new life with her hands. She was finding her own way, her own path, and I thanked God for that.

With the best of intentions I offered that woman a book and a tape, and she did not want them. We are free and even God himself respects that. Left to herself she asked for what she knew would be therapeutic for her – a needle and thread.

## SOME YEARS LATER

After surgery for secondaries, the interval between my routine medical check-ups was stretched from one month to three months to six months to twelve months. Within five years the surgeon told me that I did not require any more regular check-ups. He said, 'You are one of the lucky ones.' I was delighted on hearing this news.

For me, healing has not been something that happened suddenly, say one Wednesday afternoon at 3 p.m. It has been a lifelong process. It has been a matter of growing and maturing. And it has involved inner healing as well as a healing of the cancer. It assumed an urgency the day I was told I had cancer and in these pages I have tried to share some of the process.

I found it therapeutic to tell my friends. I felt that if they knew the truth they would help, silently but effectively, to see me through to victory. I needed their help. They were ready to help. Surely this is what is meant by Church. We cannot make it alone.

I have never liked the expression you often hear, that someone 'is fighting cancer'. This seems to imply that the person is warring against that part of themselves that is wounded, thus depleting and dividing their strength. This idea does not appeal to me. I prefer that we would look with compassion on our wounded self in order to transform it and so transcend ourselves. The doctors take care of the physical manifestation of cancer through surgery and/or other treatment. The best they can do is buy time for us to heal ourselves. And how do we heal ourselves? Each person, being unique, finds an individual path to healing. My path has been an effort to respond to a call in faith to grow deep enough spiritually to be able to contain and absorb it. Its roots are deep but the human spirit, linked to the Holy Spirit, is infinitely deeper. In my anguish I discovered that 'there is no pit so deep that He is not deeper still'; that in order to be healed *of* cancer I first had to be healed *by* cancer.

It seems that it sometimes takes a crisis such as a life-threatening illness to shock us into going down into the deepest recesses of our inmost being to accept, understand and embrace with compassion BOTH the light and the dark sides of ourselves. It is in doing so that we discover the mystery that is at the heart of us – the mystery of God himself – Emmanuel; God with us.

To be healed of cancer I first had to be healed of my dread of the thorny side of life; of my avoidance of pain at all costs; and, above all, of my denial of the dark and negative side of life. My inward journey has brought me to a place where I can now see each person as mystery –

full of light and darkness, of strength and weakness, of love and fear. The saint and the broken person can co-exist in each one of us, and life is a call to embrace them both with compassion, not only in others but above all in myself. It is only then that they can co-exist without that life-denying tension that is so destructive.

It has been a gradual and painful process for me to come to acknowledge, with maternal love, the broken part of myself. Yet, from my own experience, I now know that through acceptance of our wounds we can be healed.

Life calls us to say Amen! to the whole of our reality, and in so doing, to become whole.

## CONCLUSION: JANUARY 2010

It is now almost twenty-four years since cancer paid me a visit. The day I was told I had cancer, the bottom fell out of my world, as I knew it, only to come together again gradually at a deeper level.

Grace sometimes comes in the form of a negative. What we perceive to be the worst thing to happen in our life may turn out to be the best thing. By giving the Wounded Child in me permission to talk and express herself clearly, I reclaimed the power that had been locked into her silence. I was now listening to her voice, unlocking her emotions, acknowledging the depth of who I truly am and embracing all of me. I was liberating my whole self. During this healing process the Wounded

Child became my Angel of Light. It was from her I learned, slowly but surely, how to survive in this world and how to transcend it.

Life is all about forgiveness and letting go, but it takes time to process anguish and heartbreak. It may seem impossible to forgive someone who has seriously wronged you because to do so would imply that what they actually did wrong is okay. With insight comes the grace to accept people as they are; to choose those who are good for us and to bless and release those who are not. In my own experience, it was from this space of inner freedom that my 'angry heartbreak' was transmuted by an insight coming from a deeper place within. With this revelation came compassion and peace. Peace is the name of the Divine Physician which heals – from within.

Gradually I emerged from my journey through cancer feeling far more real and secure in the source of my own being. In other words, I was now living from the ground of my own innermost truth. Cancer woke me up to the importance of acknowledging and integrating my wounded self, enabling me to access the healing power rooted in the core of my being – my Real Self.